Reversing Morton's Neuroma: Overcoming Cravings

The Raw Vegan Plant-Based Detoxification & Regeneration Workbook for Healing Patients.

Volume 3

Health Central

Copyright © 2023

All rights reserved. Without limiting rights under the copyright reserved above, no part of this publication may be reproduced, stored, introduced into a retrieval system, distributed or transmitted in any form or by any means, including without limitation photocopying, recording, or other electronic or mechanical methods, without the prior written permission of the publisher, except in the case of brief quotations embodied in critical reviews and certain other non-commercial uses permitted by copyright law.

This book, with the opinions, suggestions and references made within it, is based on the author's personal experience and is for personal study and research purposes only. This program is about health and vitality, not disease. The author makes no medical claims. If you choose to use the material in this book on yourself, the author and publisher take no responsibility for your actions and decisions or the consequences thereof..

The scanning, uploading, and/or distribution of this document via the internet or via any other means without the permission of the publisher is illegal and is punishable by law. Please purchase only authorized editions and do not participate in or encourage electronic piracy of copyrightable materials

Topics Discussed & Journal Structure

1. Points Discussed In Previous Volume

2. Morton's Neuroma: Overcoming Cravings

3. Our Story

4. Important Notes for Overcoming Your Morton's Neuroma

5. The Power of Journaling

6. Daily Journal Examples

7. Frequently Asked Questions (Vol. 3)

8. 30 Day Assisted Journal Section

Points Discussed in Volume 2

1 – What to eat? The fruits and vegetables that we found to be most effective – along with herbs that will support your detoxification and regeneration.

2 – Maximising results whilst managing detoxification symptoms

3 - How to incorporate intermittent dry fasting into your routine. Remember to always listen to your body with any type of fasting.

4 – Sleep and its healing power. Ideal number of hours to sleep and when to wind down.

5 – The effectiveness of juicing and reducing the risk of fermentation.

6 – Useful herbs and supplementation

7 – Enjoying success with others and accountability partners.

Morton's Neuroma: Overcoming Cravings

Cravings! Oh Cravings...

So life is wonderful and full of vitality. Your consciousness has increased and your body's biology is balancing out as your improving health overpowers any previous conditions. Having experienced and accepted that we as human beings thrive on fruit with some vegetables for re-mineralisation - you are starting to see and feel the benefits of this regimen.

However, there are still times that you have powerful cravings for those specific foods and snacks that you have spent years consuming. Where are these cravings randomly coming from? Why do they come on so strongly? How can you overcome these cravings?

As the fruit disposes of the parasites and worms hidden away within your gut, they put up a fight because they do not want to leave – they need feeding and NOW! This manifests itself through strong cravings that can feel very challenging to overcome at times.

Parasites dislike energy and Oxygen - therefore they thrive on foods that have zero electromagnetic energy, with their favourites being cooked fats, starches, dairy and meat products. Fruit is nourishing life-giving food which comes with an un-matched detoxifying power and it is loaded with energy. Parasites struggle to adapt to a fruit diet hence why they trigger cravings.

Throughout our work, Fructose (fruit sugar) has worked well in the removal of parasites and cleansing of the gut. The addition of herbs can support this but in general, fruit alone is highly capable of performing well. You should see results within two to three weeks. Cravings will strike within this period - just remind yourself that this is a sign of the parasites passing away. As you alkalize and hydrate your body, the parasites will be struggling to survive so be sure to push through these feelings and keep moving forward with your protocol.

Parasites struggle to stay alive also with a diet rich in leafy green vegetables because they contain chlorophyll and this is full of electricity and Oxygen. However, fruit is far more hydrating and therefore much more effective.

If you are finding that your cravings are unbearable – then it would be wise to get yourself some herbs to assist you. Herbs that we have found to be helpful include: clove, wormwood, and black walnut. We also found specific raw foods to be satiating such as ripened bananas, dates, figs, coconut water. This will vary between individuals so you are welcome to experiment and find what works best for you.

Remove social triggers and situations that increase your desire for cooked/low energy foods. For example, we have found that previously we would find ourselves eating cooked foods more so during events, or friends/family gatherings. Be mindful of this and perhaps have a fruit salad prepared beforehand. You could also work towards showing your circle of friends and family the benefits that this protocol brings so they could also potentially join you. Getting yourself an accountability partner works well too – you can all support each other regardless of your conditions and stages. In the end, we found the underlying issues to always be the same (congestion).

Another very useful technique to become more conscious, mindful and present is to meditate. We adopted a variety of meditation methods when we were struggling to overcome strong craving attacks. A simple routine would be to calm your breathing down, relax, and focus on imagining a healing and soothing light enter into your body through your head – feel it nourish and untangle any blocked energy or resistance within that is causing these cravings to want to take over. Let this glowing light channel out all negative and non-productive thoughts and feelings – far, far out of your body through your finger tips and toes – with every calm breath you breath out, feel these cravings leave your body. This is one tried and tested routine that we have found to work with addictive behavioural patterns. Give it a try and feel the presence and calmness within. Deep, calm and rhythmical breathing contributes to this greatly.

Once you get through the early stages of your raw vegan diet routine, the chemistry within your body will start to change and you will begin noticing that you are attracted more to the beautiful and differing colours of fruits (and vegetables). Your consciousness will increase further towards nature and fellow humans. We have seen members of our community go from eating and craving chocolate daily to removing their cravings and re-channelling these feels more towards sweet tree-ripened fruits such as mangos, blueberries, strawberries, dates, etc.

Fruits will elevate your consciousness to a higher state whilst cooked foods will numb and suppress your progress. A fruit-based diet will make you face your daily challenges head on and work through them, as opposed to cooked foods which will drain you of energy, contribute towards a slower mentality and make you put off tasks to another day. Cooked foods will contribute towards holding you back, and stop you from healing, and becoming stronger as a person, both mentally and physically. Above all, you owe it to yourself to supercharge your health so that you can experience a new, enhanced you.

The major positive is that fruit is generally available in abundance – you could even grow some yourself – it is very sustainable - and providing it has been picked ripe, you will get to experience the taste of truly satisfying sweetness that will heal you whilst starving out and removing all unwanted parasites.

If you give into your cravings – you will set yourself back and if you continue to feed your parasites / fungus / worms – they will continue to live and breed within your body's environment. Just like human-beings, parasites defecate – but they don't have a bathroom, so your struggling body ends up being the victim of their waste matter. This leads to an increase in your toxic load and the creation of uric acid in the body. With yet more acids to contend with, your inflammation levels increase – leading to increased irritation and mental imbalances.

It is actually very easy to detoxify and heal yourself. YOU CAN DO THIS – just stay strong and blast these creatures out of your system with fruit (and green juices).

Having eaten cooked foods for the majority of your lifetime, it can be challenging to move over to a predominantly fruit diet, and this is why we recommend a transition period which involves the allowance of steamed starch-free vegetables, dried fruit (dates, figs, mango, raisins), avocados, bananas, tasty salads, vegetable broth – for dinner. Providing you are eating fruit during the daytime, you can follow this regimen for as long as you can feel yourself improving and growing within this routine. Ensure you load up on the fruit before dinner time, so you feel full and satisfied by the end of the day.

We recommend steamed vegetables and salads for dinner/evening time mainly because this is when the parasites tend to strike. They feed in the evenings because they prefer to come out during darkness instead of daylight. The majority of patients that we worked with also reported cravings during the evening to night time periods.

Hunger is another important topic to address. If you are hungry – this is normally a sign that you are not eating enough fruit / not consuming sufficient calories. With fruit being so much lower in calories in comparison to dense cooked food, you have to eat much more of it in order to reach your individual caloric requirement. A couple of pieces will not suffice – you will need a significant volume in order to feel satiated and carry yourself over to your next meal time. We found that caloric intake plays a significant role in feeling satiated and satisfied. Eat until your heart is content, and always focus on how your body is feeling.

In the early stages, you could over-indulge during your fruit meal times and as you improve, you can adjust this accordingly. We were never worried about over-consuming raw vegan fruit/vegetables due to them being natural and so easily digested by our bodies. The added benefit is that fruit / fructose (fruit sugar) is alive and alkaline unlike processed sugar which is acid-forming to the body.

If your body is struggling to process fructose (resulting in sudden weight gain), this could potentially point towards congestion within your adrenal glands. Once these have been cleansed and the toxic acids within your body have moved out, you will thrive on fruits. As soon as you adjust to the fruits that were intended for you by nature, eating mucus-forming / cooked starchy foods will just leave you with extreme fatigue/sleepiness because your body will struggle to come down from vitality-rich fruits and vegetables - to process and digest these low energy foods that were never meant for it. After a while on this protocol, you may find yourself becoming sensitive to acid-forming foods and your body's reaction to them will tell you everything you need to know.

Note: We have found cravings to also be a result of emotional imbalances and "comfort eating". If you have weak adrenal glands, then you may suffer from this. In this case, the focus should be on un-clogging your adrenal glands (and all related pathways/organs) through herbs (ashwagandha, licorice root, rhodiola rosea), intermittent fasting and fruit – and transitioning you gently into a longer-term detoxification (and regeneration) protocol.

Are you ready to become enlightened and move to a higher state of consciousness whilst reversing your conditions? Do you want to be free of anxiety, prolonged sadness and depression? Gift yourself with vibrant health and spiritual evolution – get back to nature and connect with the foods that were made for us to thrive on.

Our goal throughout this workbook and journal is to help you with recording your progress and applying the information stated in these sections.

Start with what you are most comfortable with and make it enjoyable, choose your favourite sweet fruits. If you deviate from the routine, we advise to get back on track as soon as possible. Just keep moving forward, keep track of progress, and be persistent.

We would like to wish you all the best. Good luck with your healing journey.

Our Story

It was a Sunday night, over 7 years ago – I was in bed – tossing and turning – unable to sleep. I watched the time pass, from 11pm, to 12am… to 1:30am. I just couldn't sleep. I could feel an immense pressure in my chest cavity and all across my diaphragm area. I couldn't understand where this was coming from. I got up and had some water, I then tried to use the bathroom – the discomfort was still there. Nothing seemed to work – I felt like I was being suffocated each time I would lie down. In the end, I fell asleep out of sheer fatigue.

At the time, I was a sufferer of asthma, eczema, anxiety attacks, and a damaged/leaky gut. These conditions had lead to many symptoms that doctors could not offer me any answers for. I had many tests done but nothing could tell me what the root causes of my problems were.

I started researching about my symptoms, and as I did this, I found myself expanding into the area of medical history. As my research continued, I came to understand that our ancestors lived healthy and long lives, without the health challenges of today.

Eventually, I stumbled upon a few health forums which I joined. Through these, I met a series of individuals that were battling a variety of conditions themselves (a rare genetic disorder, Crohn's disease, multiple sclerosis, muscular dystrophy (MD), diabetes, cushing's disease, a series of 'incurable' autoimmune diseases, and cancer).

We all came together and as we started to grow as a group, we made a significant discovery - that actually the cure to all diseases was discovered back in the 1920s by a Dr Arnold Ehret.

As we studied his material, we started applying his information and protocols on ourselves. This seemed like one experiment worth trying, and within 2 weeks, regardless of our individual conditions, we all started to notice a difference in our improved digestion, higher energy levels, increased mental clarity and improved physical ability. A major change was taking place – our health was improving, as our conditions were decreasing.

We continued to expand our knowledge and we started to encounter even more communities and learnt that there were more magnificent and very gifted healers out there. We came across the works and achievements of Dr Sebi, and completed an insightful and very informative course by Dr Robert Morse.

The essential message of these great healers was very similar to that of Dr Arnold Ehret. Now we had even further confirmation that the information we had been following thus far was in fact THE path to health success. With our progress so far, we could sense victory.

Within 3 months, 30 to 40 percent of our symptoms had disappeared and our health was becoming stronger. Some of us started to take specific herbs in order to enhance the detoxification.

Another 3 months on and the majority of us no longer experienced any more symptoms. Our blood work had also improved significantly, but we still had work to do in order to completely heal.

Now that we had made significant progress in reversing our conditions through self-experimentation, we started to offer basic healthy eating advice to the sick within our local communities.

Eventually, we started working with local patients on a voluntary basis. It was heartbreaking to witness lives being cut short or chronic sickness being accepted as a way of life – all whilst the lifelong eating habits of these individuals remained. The most common diseases that we were coming across included: cancers, heart disease, chronic kidney disease, high blood pressure, varying infections, and diabetes.

By helping our communities with changing their daily eating habits, we started seeing results, and although the transitional phase of moving from the foods that they were so used to eating, to moving over to a raw plant-based routine was a challenge, in the end, it was worth the shift. Note: there were many that ignored our advice and sadly they continued to remain in their state.

We did have resistance initially from family members and friends of the sick but after some time as they started seeing health improvements, more started joining us, and they also started experiencing what we had when we first set out on our journey of natural self-healing.

Nevertheless, challenges still remained – the main ones being the undoing of society's programming that cooked food is an essential part of life (including animal and wheat based products) and raw food alone surely cannot be good for you. It doesn't take long to explain how to remove imbalances and dis-ease from within the human body but the more extensive task is to actually have the protocol information applied and adhered to completely.

This is where the idea for this series of journal & progress tracker stemmed from. We felt compelled to spread this information in a more digestible and applicable form, over a series of volumes, in which we would start by offering some key informative points, followed by a journal which would allow for you to actually apply the information, record your progress, daily feelings and stay accountable to yourself. We also found that journaling and writing to oneself really helps to self-motivate and enhances a self consciousness that is needed when following a protocol like this.

Each journal volume within this series will be designed to help you record your journey for a 30 day period. At the start of each journal we will continue to offer insightful information about our experiences, whilst expanding on and re-iterating specific parts of this protocol.

The fact that you are reading this foreword is an indication that you are already on your way to self-healing. Regardless of your condition, we invite you to seek more knowledge and set your health free.

May you always remain blessed and guided.

Much Love From The Health Central Team

Important Notes for Overcoming Your Morton's Neuroma

1. It should be noted that based on our experiences and understanding, whether your condition is Morton's Neuroma, or any other, we recommend the same raw vegan healing protocol across all spectrums. With some conditions, you may need to perform a deeper detoxification (using herbs - or organ/glandular meat/capsules for more chronic situations) before achieving significant results, but in general, we have found this protocol to work in most cases. In our experience, the goal is not to cure, but instead to raise health levels first, through healthy food choices, as intended for our species – before the eradication and prevention of these modern-day "disease" conditions can take place.

2. With all conditions, we have found that the lymphatic system has become congested and overwhelmed due to the kidneys not efficiently filtering out the accumulated cell waste – as a result of years of dehydrating cooked/wheat/dairy foods. The adrenal glands work closely with the kidneys, and so adrenal/kidney herbs and glandular formulas played a major role in opening up these channels. We also found that opening up the bowels and loosening the gut was hugely important too.

3. The healing protocol that we used on ourselves is discussed and expanded upon throughout the various volumes in this series. Our goal is to share information that we have gathered from our journeys, and let you decide if it is something that you feel could also work for you in your

journey for health and vitality. You are not obliged to use this information, and you may proceed as you see fit.

Through our study, research and application, we have found this system to correct any internal imbalances and remove dis-ease that has occurred within the human body, due to the continued consumption of acid-forming foods.

4. Always take progression ultra slow and go at your own pace. Listen to your body at every stage. We cannot re-iterate this point enough. Pay attention to how you feel and continue to consult your doctor and monitor your blood work.

5. A special emphasis needs to be given to the transition phase when moving from your regular, standard diet, to a raw vegan diet that is high in fruit. You must take your time and slowly remove foods from your current routine, and replace them with either fasting or a small amount of fruit in the initial stages. Work with small amounts – please do not make any drastic changes. If you do not feel comfortable or have any concerns at any stage, please immediately stop.

Note: with any dietary change, this can be a stressful event for the body and so it is important that you support your kidneys and adrenal glands using the appropriate herbs and glandular formulas previously mentioned.

6. Before partaking in any new dietary routine, please always consult your Doctor first and ensure that they are aware of your health related goals. This approach is beneficial because (a) you can monitor your blood work with your doctor as you progress with this new protocol, and (b) if you are on any medication, as your health improves, you

can review its need and/or discuss having dosage amounts reduced (if necessary).

7. Please note that we are sharing information from our collective experiences of how we healed ourselves from a variety of diseases and conditions. These are solely our own opinions. Having reversed a range of conditions using essentially the same protocol, our understanding and conclusion, based on our experience alone, is that regardless of the disease, illness or condition name – removing it from the human body stems from correcting your diet and transitioning over to a more raw vegan lifestyle.

8. Proceed with care, and again, do not make any sudden changes – always take your time in slowly removing foods that are not serving you, and replacing them with high energy sweet tree-ripened juicy fruit. If at any point you feel that you are moving too quickly, please adjust your transition accordingly. Results may vary between individuals.

9. We recommended that you constantly expand your knowledge and familiarise yourself with the works of Dr Arnold Ehret, Dr Robert Morse and John Rose. When you feel confident with your understanding, start taking gradual steps towards reaching your goals. Make the most of this journal and use it to serve you as a companion on your journey.

The Power of Journaling

a) Journaling your inner self talk is a truly effective way of increasing self awareness and consciousness. To be able to transfer your thoughts and feelings onto a piece of paper is a truly effective method of self reflection and improvement. This is much needed when you are switching to a high fruit dietary routine.

b) Be sure to always add the date of journaling at the top of each page used. This is invaluable for when you wish to go back and review/track progress and your feelings/thoughts on previous dates.

c) Keep a comprehensive record of activities, thoughts, and really log everything you ate/are eating. You can even make miscellaneous notes if you feel that they will help you.

d) We have added tips and questions to offer you guidance, reminders, inspiration and areas to journal about.

e) We like to use journals to have a conversation with ourselves. Inner talk can really help you overcome any challenges that you are experiencing. Express yourself and any concerns that you may have.

f) Try to advise yourself as though you are your best friend – similarly to how you would advise a close friend or family member. You will be surprised at the results that you will achieve from using this technique.

g) Add notes to this journal and work your way through the 30 days. Once completed, move onto the next journal volume in this series, which will also be structured in a similar, supportive and educational fashion. We have produced a series of these journals in order to cater for your ongoing journey and goals.

h) For those of you who would like to track your progress with a more basic notebook-style journal, we have produced a separate series in which each notebook interior differs. This is to cater for your complete health journaling needs.

We have laid out the following examples to serve as potential frameworks for one way of how a journal could be filled in on a daily basis. These are just basic examples, but you can complete your daily journals in any other way that you feel is most comfortable and effective for you.

[EXAMPLE 1]
Today's Date: 2nd Jan 2020

Morning
I just ate 3 mangoes - very sweet and tasty. I felt a heavy feeling under my chest area so I stopped eating. Unsure what that was - maybe digestive or the transverse colon?

Afternoon
I was feeling hungry so I am eating some dried figs, pineapple and apricots with around 750ml of spring water.

Evening
Sipping on a green tea (herbal). Feeling pretty strong and alert at the moment.

Night
Enjoying a bowl of red seeded grapes. Currently I feel satisfied.

Today's Notes (Highlights, Thoughts, Feelings):

Unlike yesterday, today was a good day. I am noticing an increase in regular bowel movements which makes me feel cleansed and light afterwards. I feel as though my kidneys are also starting to filter better (white sediment visible in morning wee).

It definitely helps to document my thoughts in this workbook. A great way to reflect, improve and stay on track.

Feeling very good - vibrant and strong - I have noticed a major improvement in my physical fitness and performance. Mentally I feel healthier and happier.

[EXAMPLE 2]
Today's Date: 3rd Jan 2020

Morning
Dry fasting (water and food free since 8pm last night) - will go up until 12:30pm today, and start with 500ml of spring water before eating half a watermelon.

Afternoon
Kept busy and was in and out quite a bit – so nothing consumed.

Evening
At around 5pm, I had a peppermint tea with a selection of mixed dried fruit (small bowl of apricot, dates, mango, pineapple, and prunes).

Night
Sipped on spring water through the evening as required.
Finished off the other half of the watermelon from the morning.

Today's Notes (Highlights, Thoughts, Feelings):

As with most days, today started well with me dry fasting (continuing my fast from my sleep/skipping breakfast) up until around 12:30pm and then eating half a watermelon. The laxative effect of the watermelon helped me poop and release any loosened toxins from the fasting period.
I tend to struggle on some days from 3pm onwards. Up until that point I am okay but if the cravings strike then it can be challenging. I remind myself that those burgers and chips do not have any live healing energy.
I feel good in general. I feel fantastic doing a fruit/juice fast but slightly empty by the end of the day.
Cooked food makes me feel severe fatigue and mental fog.
Will continue with my fruit fasting and start to introduce fruit juices due to their deeper detox benefits. I would love to be on juices only as I have seen others within the community achieve amazing results.

[EXAMPLE 3]
Today's Date: 4th Jan 2020

Morning
Today I woke and my children were enjoying some watermelon for breakfast – and the smell was luring so I joined them. Large bowl of watermelon eaten at around 8am. Started with a glass of water.

Afternoon
Snacked on left over watermelon throughout the morning and afternoon. Had 5 dates an hour or so after.

Evening
Had around 3 mangoes at around 6pm. Felt content – but then I was invited round to a family gathering where a selection of pizzas, burgers and chips were being served. I gave into the peer pressure and felt like I let myself down!

Night
Having over-eaten earlier on in the evening, I was still feeling bloated with a headache (possibly digestion related) and I also felt quite mucus filled (wheez in chest and coughing up phlegm). Very sleepy and low energy. The perils of cooked foods!!

Today's Notes (Highlights, Thoughts, Feelings):

I let myself down today. It all started well until I ate a fully blown meal (and over-ate). I didn't remain focussed and I spun off track. As a result my energy levels were much lower and I felt a bout of extreme fatigue 30 minutes after the meal (most likely the body struggling to with digesting all that cooked food).
I need to stick to the plan because the difference between fruit fasting, and eating cooked foods is huge – 1 makes you feel empowered whilst the other makes you feel drained. I also felt the mucus overload after the meal – it kicked in pretty quickly.
Today I felt disappointed after giving in to the meal but tomorrow is a new day and I will keep on going! It is important to remind myself that I won't get better if I cannot stick to the routine.

Frequently Asked Questions (Vol. 3)

Can I spray vitamin B12 (and other vitamins/minerals/supplements) onto my fruit?

You could do, if you are heavily deficient in the initial stages. Within the broad range of fruits available today, you will find all nutrients present (all biologically available and easily absorbed by the body). This raw diet is far superior to anything else out there as it was originally intended for the human body. If you initially have deficiencies then you may opt to use supplementation but with time, as your body normalises/detoxifies and adapts, you will find that you will no longer be deficient in anything, and your absorption of nutrients from food will also return (all of our patients initially suffer from mal-absorption due to congestion in the gut).

It is hard for me to dry fast as I get thirsty regularly. Is it okay for me to do a water fast?

Water fasting works well and you will find great benefit in this. You could even slow juice your fruit (and some vegetables if needed) and perform a fast purely on juiced fruit - this would be more powerful. Many within the Fruitarian community talk about this and the "solid food vacation". Do try to work your way up to dry fasting (hint: you dry fast during sleep). Be sure to support your kidneys and adrenal glands with either herbs or kidney and adrenal glandular capsules because the toxic load leaving your body via your skin, and kidneys will be highly concentrated in acidity and could knock them harshly - so be aware of this.

How am I supposed to stay full on an all-fruit diet?

We don't recommend just jumping straight into an all-fruit diet immediately. During the transition stages of moving from cooked foods to a fruit diet, we recommend that you increase your fruit intake each time you feel hungry and in addition make a large salad to serve as a filler. The salad could consist of lettuce, any leafy greens, tomatoes, cucumber, onions, sweet-corn, mushrooms, avocado (mashed up as the sauce), lemon juice, and even some optional tahini (crushed sesame seed paste). This is just one sample recipe – there are many ways to make a delicious salad. Many choose to also make a variety of raw zucchini spaghetti dishes with the sauce being made of blended tomatoes, sun-dried tomatoes, basil, onions and a dash of garlic. Again, this is just one example – with research, you will discover many more tasty recipes that can really support you in the transition phase. Always aim to return to fruit – this should be your default diet.

30 Day Assisted Journal Section

1. Today's Date:

Morning
(work towards continuing your night time dry fast up until at least 12pm)

Afternoon
(get hydrating with fresh fruit or even better slow juiced fruits/berries/melons)

Evening
(aim to wind down to a dry fast by around 6pm to 7pm)

Night
(work your way up to dry fasting from the evening until 12pm the following day)

Today's Notes (Highlights, Thoughts, Feelings, What Could You Improve On?)

"Keep a positive mindset. Remind yourself that everything is possible & you WILL achieve your goals"

2. Today's Date:

Morning
(work towards continuing your night time dry fast up until at least 12pm)

Afternoon
(get hydrating with fresh fruit or even better slow juiced fruits/berries/melons)

Evening
(aim to wind down to a dry fast by around 6pm to 7pm)

Night
(work your way up to dry fasting from the evening until 12pm the following day)

Today's Notes (Highlights, Thoughts, Feelings, What Could You Improve On?)

"Sleep is very vital for your healing. Wind down by 7pm and aim to be in bed by 10pm to 10:30pm (if possible)."

3. Today's Date:

Morning
(work towards continuing your night time dry fast up until at least 12pm)

Afternoon
(get hydrating with fresh fruit or even better slow juiced fruits/berries/melons)

Evening
(aim to wind down to a dry fast by around 6pm to 7pm)

Night
(work your way up to dry fasting from the evening until 12pm the following day)

Today's Notes (Highlights, Thoughts, Feelings, What Could You Improve On?)

"Eat melons/watermelons separately, and before any other fruit as it digests faster and we want to limit fermentation (acidity) which can occur if other fruits are mixed in."

4. Today's Date:

Morning
(work towards continuing your night time dry fast up until at least 12pm)

Afternoon
(get hydrating with fresh fruit or even better slow juiced fruits/berries/melons)

Evening
(aim to wind down to a dry fast by around 6pm to 7pm)

Night
(work your way up to dry fasting from the evening until 12pm the following day)

Today's Notes (Highlights, Thoughts, Feelings, What Could You Improve On?)

"Use parsley to support kidney filtration & to detox mercury out of your body."

5. Today's Date:

Morning
(work towards continuing your night time dry fast up until at least 12pm)

Afternoon
(get hydrating with fresh fruit or even better slow juiced fruits/berries/melons)

Evening
(aim to wind down to a dry fast by around 6pm to 7pm)

Night
(work your way up to dry fasting from the evening until 12pm the following day)

Today's Notes (Highlights, Thoughts, Feelings, What Could You Improve On?)

"Meditate and perform deep breathing exercises in order to help yourself remain present minded and stay on track."

6. Today's Date:

Morning
(work towards continuing your night time dry fast up until at least 12pm)

Afternoon
(get hydrating with fresh fruit or even better slow juiced fruits/berries/melons)

Evening
(aim to wind down to a dry fast by around 6pm to 7pm)

Night
(work your way up to dry fasting from the evening until 12pm the following day)

Today's Notes (Highlights, Thoughts, Feelings, What Could You Improve On?)

"Ensure any amalgam fillings in your teeth are replaced with composite fillings – preferably by a holistic dentist."

7. Today's Date:

Morning
(work towards continuing your night time dry fast up until at least 12pm)

Afternoon
(get hydrating with fresh fruit or even better slow juiced fruits/berries/melons)

Evening
(aim to wind down to a dry fast by around 6pm to 7pm)

Night
(work your way up to dry fasting from the evening until 12pm the following day)

Today's Notes (Highlights, Thoughts, Feelings, What Could You Improve On?)

"If you are struggling with hunger pangs in the early stages, try some dates or dried apricots, prunes, or raisins, with a cup of herbal tea.

8. Today's Date:

Morning
(work towards continuing your night time dry fast up until at least 12pm)

Afternoon
(get hydrating with fresh fruit or even better slow juiced fruits/berries/melons)

Evening
(aim to wind down to a dry fast by around 6pm to 7pm)

Night
(work your way up to dry fasting from the evening until 12pm the following day)

Today's Notes (Highlights, Thoughts, Feelings, What Could You Improve On?)

"Keep on loving! Love is alkalizing, it improves digestion and kidney elimination. Your blood and lymph flow will also improve."

9. Today's Date:

Morning
(work towards continuing your night time dry fast up until at least 12pm)

Afternoon
(get hydrating with fresh fruit or even better slow juiced fruits/berries/melons)

Evening
(aim to wind down to a dry fast by around 6pm to 7pm)

Night
(work your way up to dry fasting from the evening until 12pm the following day)

Today's Notes (Highlights, Thoughts, Feelings, What Could You Improve On?)

"Regularly remind yourself about the great rewards and benefits that you will experience from keeping up this detox."

10. Today's Date:

Morning
(work towards continuing your night time dry fast up until at least 12pm)

Afternoon
(get hydrating with fresh fruit or even better slow juiced fruits/berries/melons)

Evening
(aim to wind down to a dry fast by around 6pm to 7pm)

Night
(work your way up to dry fasting from the evening until 12pm the following day)

Today's Notes (Highlights, Thoughts, Feelings, What Could You Improve On?)

"Keep your teeth brushed and flossed regularly – at least twice a day to keep them healthy for your fruit sessions. You will notice an improvement in your dental health with this raw/fruit diet."

11. Today's Date:

Morning
(work towards continuing your night time dry fast up until at least 12pm)

Afternoon
(get hydrating with fresh fruit or even better slow juiced fruits/berries/melons)

Evening
(aim to wind down to a dry fast by around 6pm to 7pm)

Night
(work your way up to dry fasting from the evening until 12pm the following day)

Today's Notes (Highlights, Thoughts, Feelings, What Could You Improve On?)

"Pain is merely a sign of energy blockage(s) resulting from acidosis. Alkalization is the key (through detoxification)."

12. Today's Date: _____

Morning
(work towards continuing your night time dry fast up until at least 12pm)

Afternoon
(get hydrating with fresh fruit or even better slow juiced fruits/berries/melons)

Evening
(aim to wind down to a dry fast by around 6pm to 7pm)

Night
(work your way up to dry fasting from the evening until 12pm the following day)

Today's Notes (Highlights, Thoughts, Feelings, What Could You Improve On?)

"Embrace your achievements and wonderful results – feel and appreciate the difference within you as a result of this new routine."

13. Today's Date:

———————————— Morning ————————————
(work towards continuing your night time dry fast up until at least 12pm)

———————————— Afternoon ————————————
(get hydrating with fresh fruit or even better slow juiced fruits/berries/melons)

———————————— Evening ————————————
(aim to wind down to a dry fast by around 6pm to 7pm)

———————————— Night ————————————
(work your way up to dry fasting from the evening until 12pm the following day)

Today's Notes (Highlights, Thoughts, Feelings, What Could You Improve On?)

"Your body can use sweating (fevers), vomiting, diarrhea, frequent urination, colds, flus, and daily elimination as means to detox a toxic state. Let it run its course."

14. Today's Date:

Morning
(work towards continuing your night time dry fast up until at least 12pm)

Afternoon
(get hydrating with fresh fruit or even better slow juiced fruits/berries/melons)

Evening
(aim to wind down to a dry fast by around 6pm to 7pm)

Night
(work your way up to dry fasting from the evening until 12pm the following day)

Today's Notes (Highlights, Thoughts, Feelings, What Could You Improve On?)

"Stay as busy as you can during the daytime. Creating a busy routine makes it easier to manage your diet."

15. Today's Date:

Morning
(work towards continuing your night time dry fast up until at least 12pm)

Afternoon
(get hydrating with fresh fruit or even better slow juiced fruits/berries/melons)

Evening
(aim to wind down to a dry fast by around 6pm to 7pm)

Night
(work your way up to dry fasting from the evening until 12pm the following day)

Today's Notes (Highlights, Thoughts, Feelings, What Could You Improve On?)

"Mucus congestion (caused by dairy products) leads to a lack of mineral utilization (Calcium, Magnesium, Potassium, etc)."

16. Today's Date:

Morning
(work towards continuing your night time dry fast up until at least 12pm)

Afternoon
(get hydrating with fresh fruit or even better slow juiced fruits/berries/melons)

Evening
(aim to wind down to a dry fast by around 6pm to 7pm)

Night
(work your way up to dry fasting from the evening until 12pm the following day)

Today's Notes (Highlights, Thoughts, Feelings, What Could You Improve On?)

"Monitor your urine regularly. Urinate in a jar and leave overnight. If you see a thick cloud of white sediment (success!), your kidneys are filtering acids out."

17. Today's Date:

Morning
(work towards continuing your night time dry fast up until at least 12pm)

Afternoon
(get hydrating with fresh fruit or even better slow juiced fruits/berries/melons)

Evening
(aim to wind down to a dry fast by around 6pm to 7pm)

Night
(work your way up to dry fasting from the evening until 12pm the following day)

Today's Notes (Highlights, Thoughts, Feelings, What Could You Improve On?)

"Fructose (the sugar found in fruits) is kind to the pancreas and its absorption into the body uses minimal energy."

18. Today's Date:

Morning
(work towards continuing your night time dry fast up until at least 12pm)

Afternoon
(get hydrating with fresh fruit or even better slow juiced fruits/berries/melons)

Evening
(aim to wind down to a dry fast by around 6pm to 7pm)

Night
(work your way up to dry fasting from the evening until 12pm the following day)

Today's Notes (Highlights, Thoughts, Feelings, What Could You Improve On?)

"Filter out unwanted acids with this alkaline water-dense fruits protocol."

19. Today's Date:

Morning
(work towards continuing your night time dry fast up until at least 12pm)

Afternoon
(get hydrating with fresh fruit or even better slow juiced fruits/berries/melons)

Evening
(aim to wind down to a dry fast by around 6pm to 7pm)

Night
(work your way up to dry fasting from the evening until 12pm the following day)

Today's Notes (Highlights, Thoughts, Feelings, What Could You Improve On?)

"Fruits will empower you, providing live energy. Cooked foods in comparison will use vital energy that could otherwise be used for healing."

20. Today's Date:

——————————————— **Morning** ———————————————

(work towards continuing your night time dry fast up until at least 12pm)

——————————————— **Afternoon** ———————————————

(get hydrating with fresh fruit or even better slow juiced fruits/berries/melons)

——————————————— **Evening** ———————————————

(aim to wind down to a dry fast by around 6pm to 7pm)

——————————————— **Night** ———————————————

(work your way up to dry fasting from the evening until 12pm the following day)

Today's Notes (Highlights, Thoughts, Feelings, What Could You Improve On?)

"Infections emerge in an acidic environment"

21. Today's Date:

Morning
(work towards continuing your night time dry fast up until at least 12pm)

Afternoon
(get hydrating with fresh fruit or even better slow juiced fruits/berries/melons)

Evening
(aim to wind down to a dry fast by around 6pm to 7pm)

Night
(work your way up to dry fasting from the evening until 12pm the following day)

Today's Notes (Highlights, Thoughts, Feelings, What Could You Improve On?)

"Disease is not the presence of something evil, but rather the lack of the presence of something essential."
— Dr. Bernard Jensen.

22. Today's Date:

Morning
(work towards continuing your night time dry fast up until at least 12pm)

Afternoon
(get hydrating with fresh fruit or even better slow juiced fruits/berries/melons)

Evening
(aim to wind down to a dry fast by around 6pm to 7pm)

Night
(work your way up to dry fasting from the evening until 12pm the following day)

Today's Notes (Highlights, Thoughts, Feelings, What Could You Improve On?)

"Dependant on how deeply you detox yourself, you could even eliminate any genetic weaknesses that you may have inherited."

23. Today's Date:

Morning
(work towards continuing your night time dry fast up until at least 12pm)

Afternoon
(get hydrating with fresh fruit or even better slow juiced fruits/berries/melons)

Evening
(aim to wind down to a dry fast by around 6pm to 7pm)

Night
(work your way up to dry fasting from the evening until 12pm the following day)

Today's Notes (Highlights, Thoughts, Feelings, What Could You Improve On?)

"Keep focused on your detox. Even past injuries / trauma are all repairable for good."

24. Today's Date:

Morning
(work towards continuing your night time dry fast up until at least 12pm)

Afternoon
(get hydrating with fresh fruit or even better slow juiced fruits/berries/melons)

Evening
(aim to wind down to a dry fast by around 6pm to 7pm)

Night
(work your way up to dry fasting from the evening until 12pm the following day)

Today's Notes (Highlights, Thoughts, Feelings, What Could You Improve On?)

"If you suffer from ongoing sadness / depression, a deep detox will support your mental health. You will soon notice a positive change in your mood."

25. Today's Date:

Morning
(work towards continuing your night time dry fast up until at least 12pm)

Afternoon
(get hydrating with fresh fruit or even better slow juiced fruits/berries/melons)

Evening
(aim to wind down to a dry fast by around 6pm to 7pm)

Night
(work your way up to dry fasting from the evening until 12pm the following day)

Today's Notes (Highlights, Thoughts, Feelings, What Could You Improve On?)

"Most people do not breathe effectively. Your body requires a healthy supply of oxygen to heal. Practice breathing techniques daily."

26. Today's Date:

Morning
(work towards continuing your night time dry fast up until at least 12pm)

Afternoon
(get hydrating with fresh fruit or even better slow juiced fruits/berries/melons)

Evening
(aim to wind down to a dry fast by around 6pm to 7pm)

Night
(work your way up to dry fasting from the evening until 12pm the following day)

Today's Notes (Highlights, Thoughts, Feelings, What Could You Improve On?)

"The kidneys dislike proteins but really appreciate juicy fruits like melons, berries, citrus fruits, pineapples, mangoes, apples, grapes."

---

27. Today's Date:

Morning
(work towards continuing your night time dry fast up until at least 12pm)

Afternoon
(get hydrating with fresh fruit or even better slow juiced fruits/berries/melons)

Evening
(aim to wind down to a dry fast by around 6pm to 7pm)

Night
(work your way up to dry fasting from the evening until 12pm the following day)

Today's Notes (Highlights, Thoughts, Feelings, What Could You Improve On?)

"If you are on medications, monitor the relevant statistics (e.g. blood pressure, blood sugar level, etc). Upon improving, lower medication"

28. Today's Date:

Morning
(work towards continuing your night time dry fast up until at least 12pm)

Afternoon
(get hydrating with fresh fruit or even better slow juiced fruits/berries/melons)

Evening
(aim to wind down to a dry fast by around 6pm to 7pm)

Night
(work your way up to dry fasting from the evening until 12pm the following day)

Today's Notes (Highlights, Thoughts, Feelings, What Could You Improve On?)

"Keep your body in an alkaline state as this is where regeneration takes place."

29. Today's Date:

Morning
(work towards continuing your night time dry fast up until at least 12pm)

Afternoon
(get hydrating with fresh fruit or even better slow juiced fruits/berries/melons)

Evening
(aim to wind down to a dry fast by around 6pm to 7pm)

Night
(work your way up to dry fasting from the evening until 12pm the following day)

Today's Notes (Highlights, Thoughts, Feelings, What Could You Improve On?)

"Your skin is the largest eliminative organ. Skin brushing and sweating are crucial. Sauna heat is ideal, steam can also work."

30. Today's Date:

Morning
(work towards continuing your night time dry fast up until at least 12pm)

Afternoon
(get hydrating with fresh fruit or even better slow juiced fruits/berries/melons)

Evening
(aim to wind down to a dry fast by around 6pm to 7pm)

Night
(work your way up to dry fasting from the evening until 12pm the following day)

Today's Notes (Highlights, Thoughts, Feelings, What Could You Improve On?)

"Have your iris' read by an iridologist that works with Dr Bernard Jensen's system."

www.ingramcontent.com/pod-product-compliance
Lightning Source LLC
Chambersburg PA
CBHW031203020426
42333CB00013B/789